My Hero Wears a Mask

A Little Miss Story

By Erica Basora

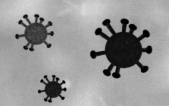
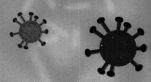

ISBN: 978-1-953751-15-7

Publisher: That's Love Publishing
Website: thatslovepublishing.com

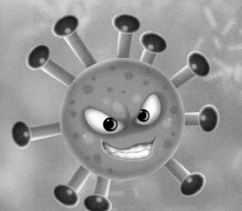
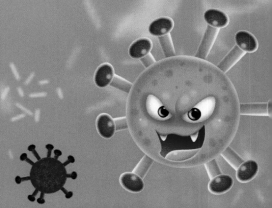

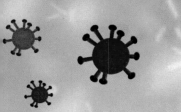

Dedication

To all essential workers. You are appreciated, you are valued, and you are loved. Thank you for providing the services needed to keep us safe and sustained. You are all our Heroes!

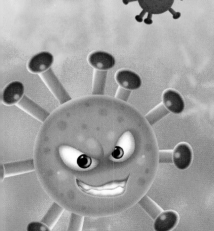
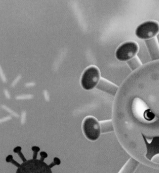
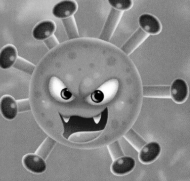

Little Miss is excited to go to school today,
There is a special announcement on the way.

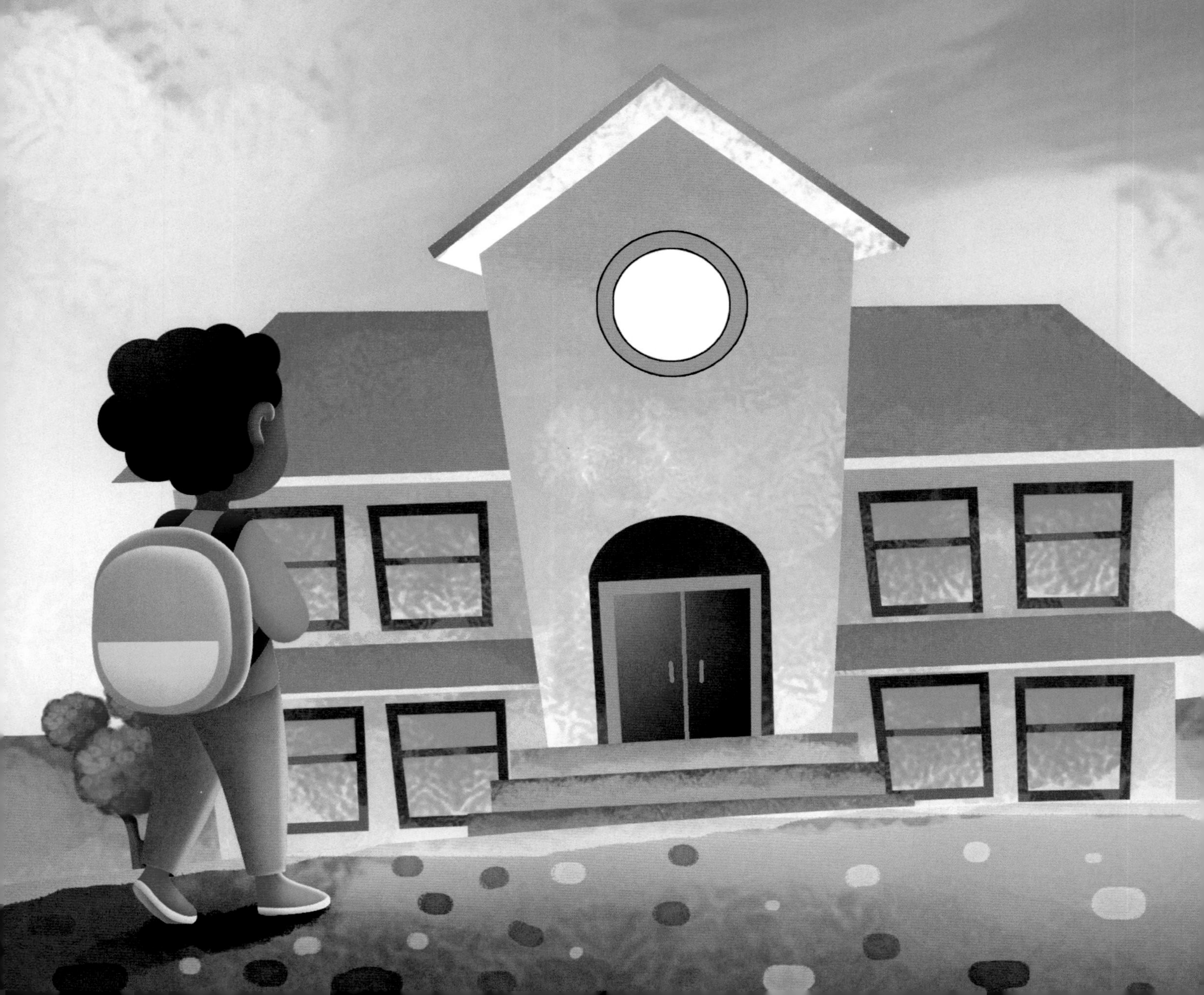

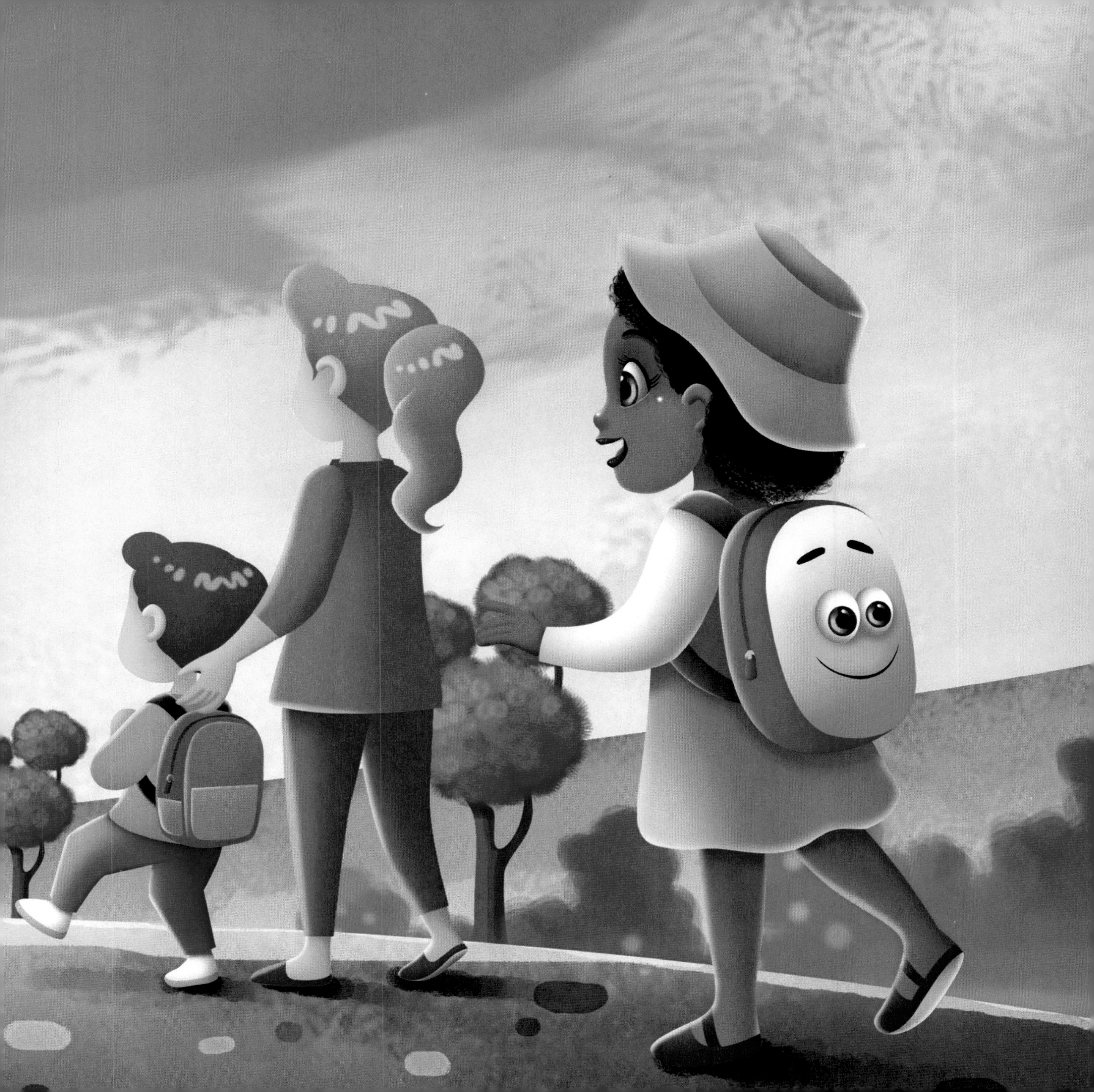

Good Morning, class!

Good Morning, Mr. Jazz!

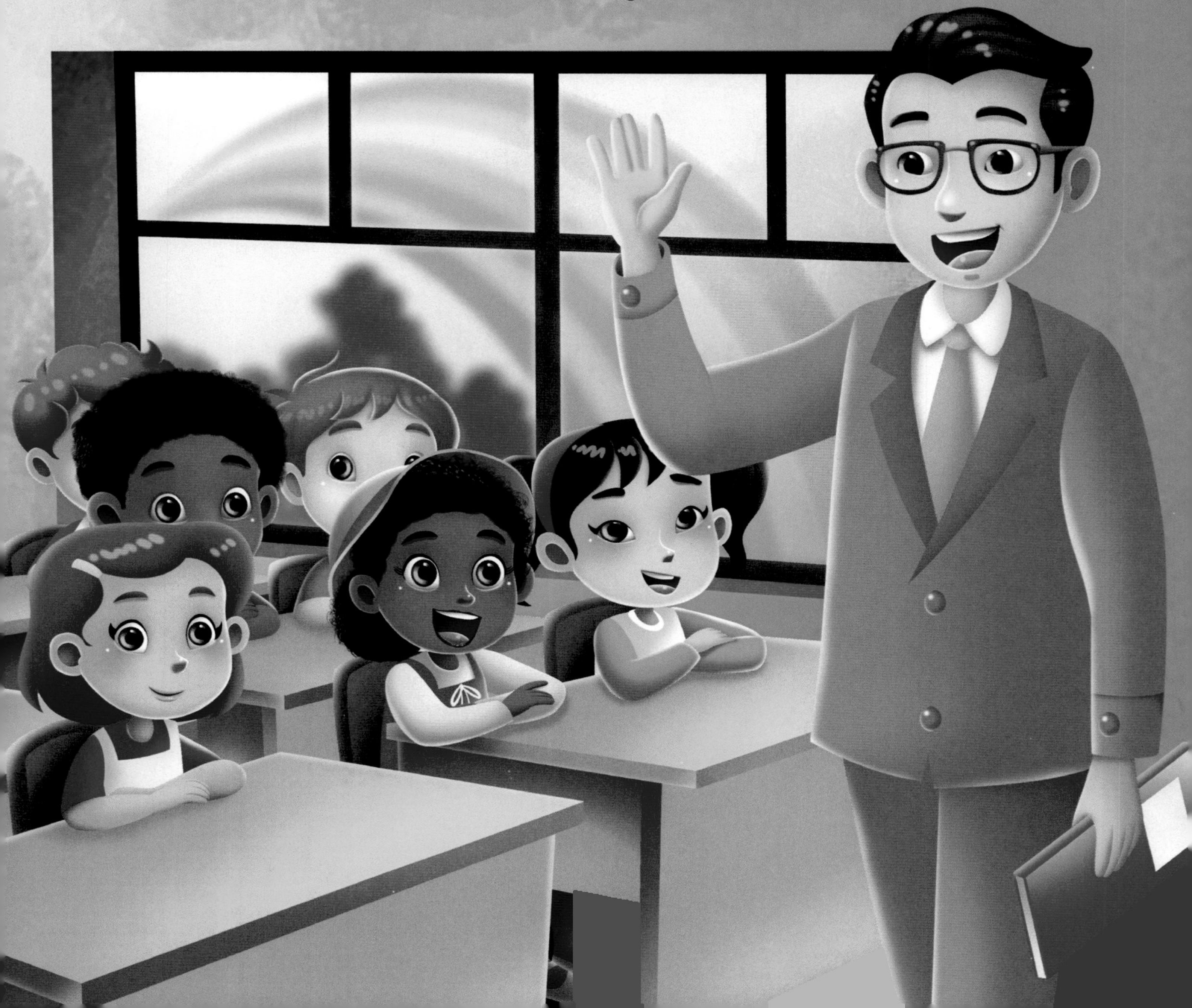

Today, we start the annual essay contest.
To see if you are chosen above the rest.

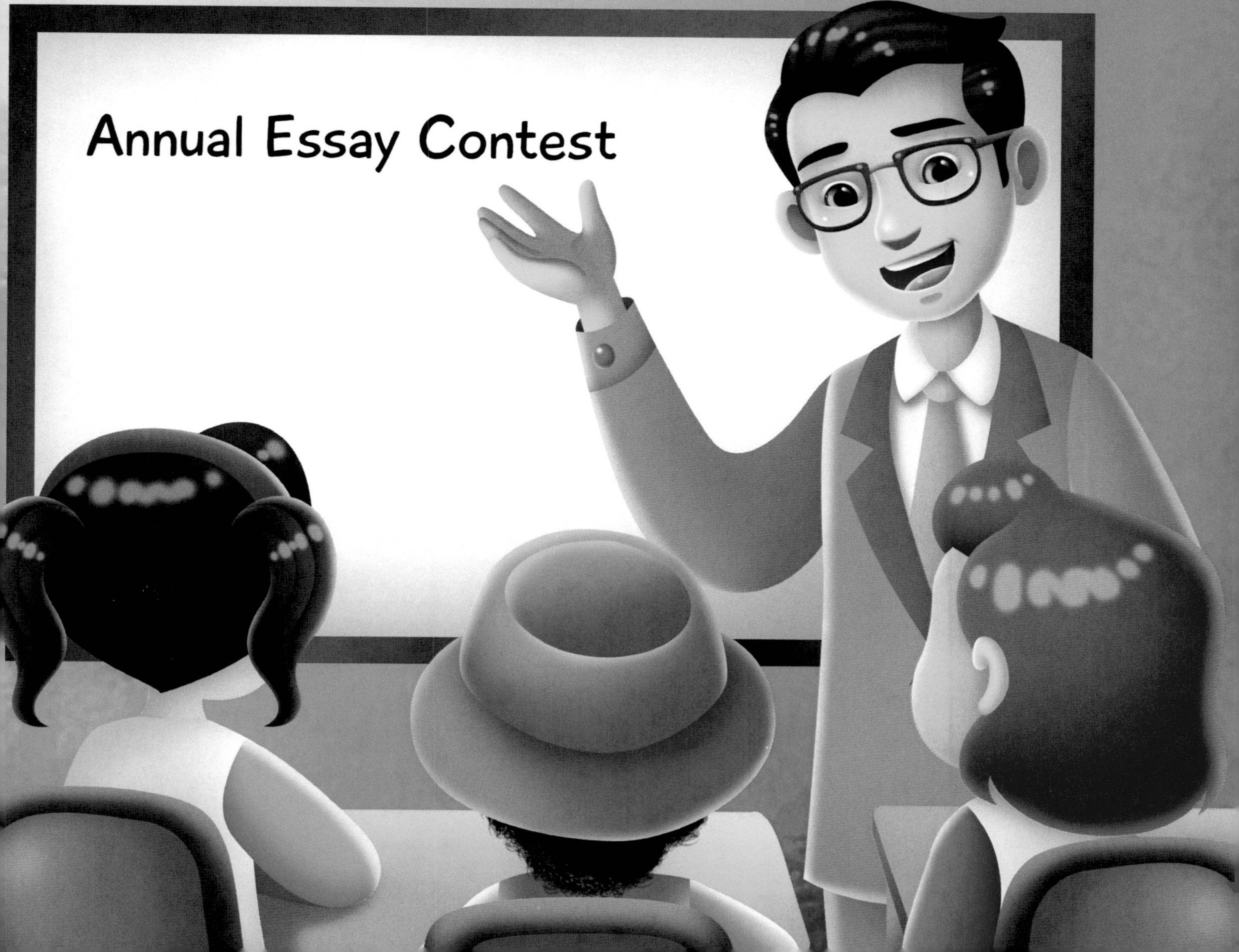
Annual Essay Contest

How excited are all of you?

Little Miss hopes hers is among the chosen few.

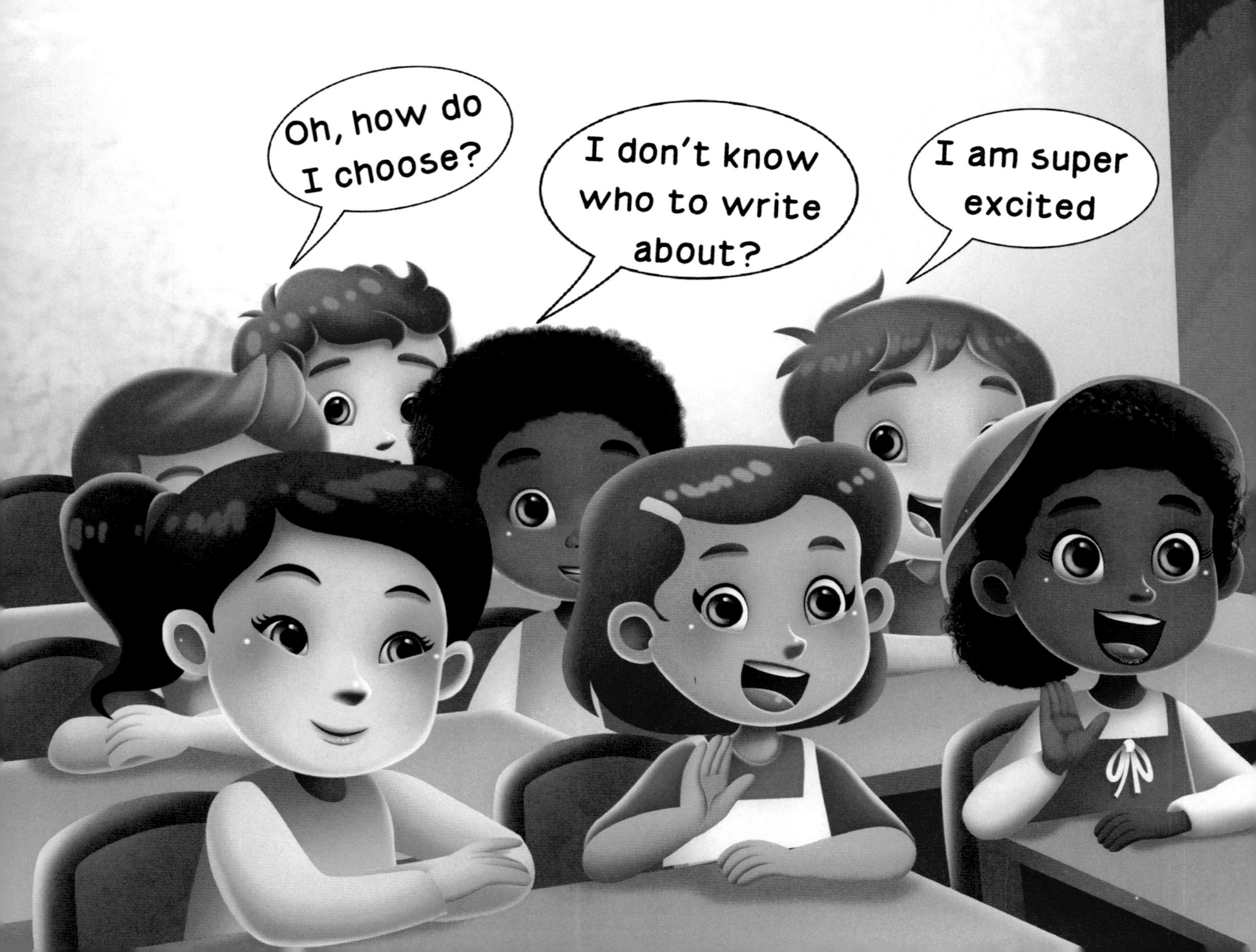
Oh, how do I choose?
I don't know who to write about?
I am super excited

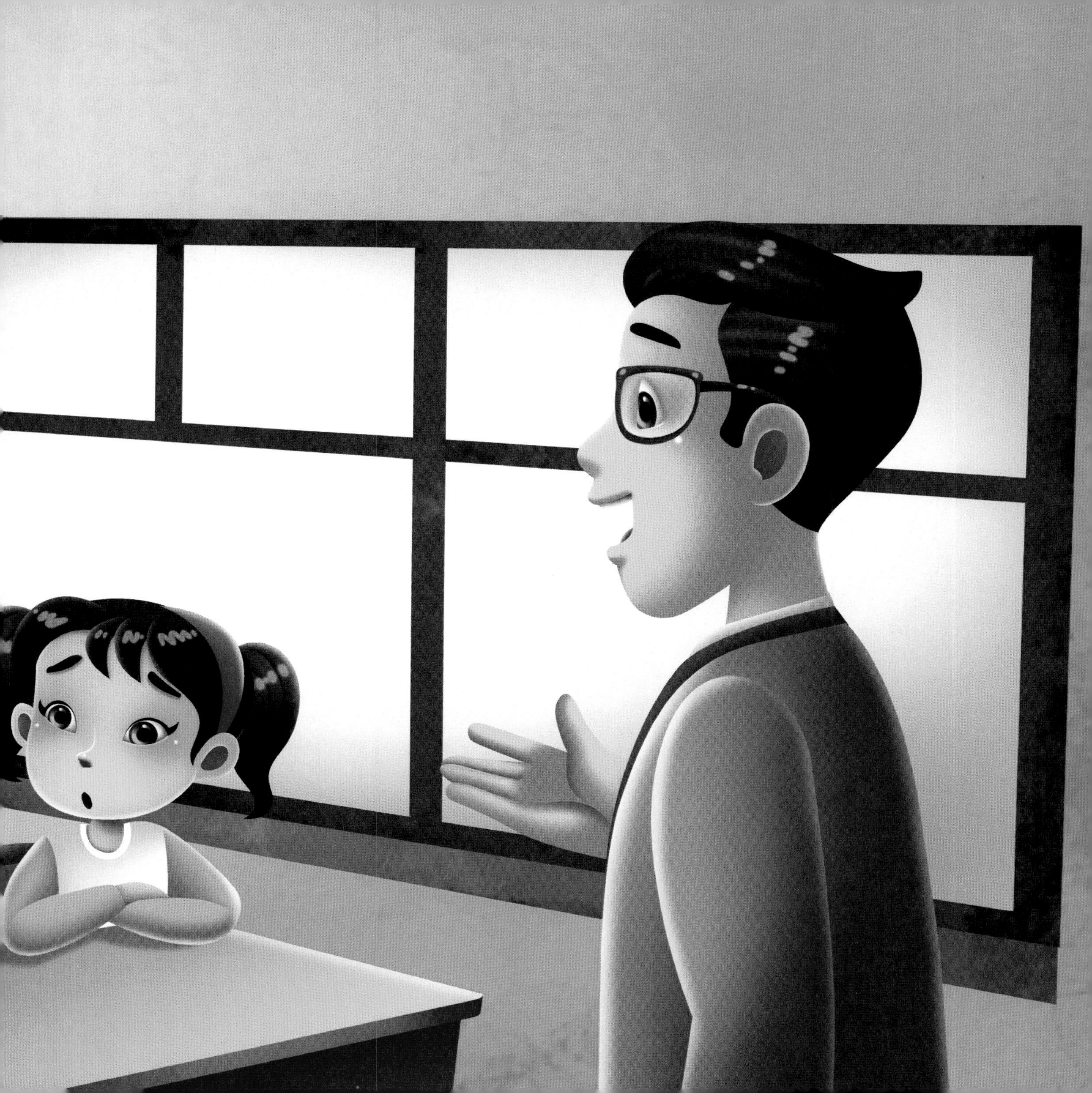

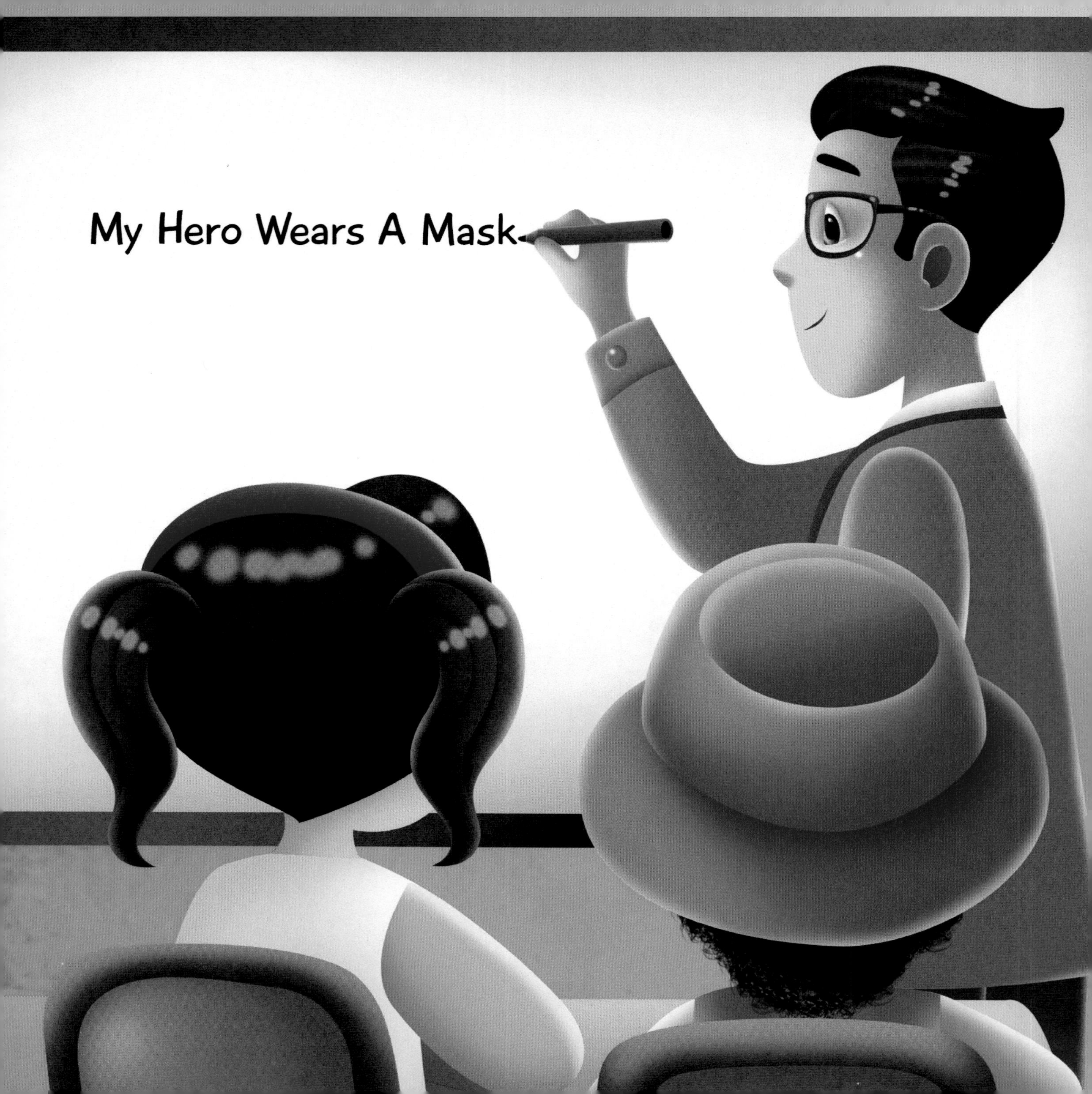
My Hero Wears A Mask

The theme this year is, MY HERO WEARS A MASK.

Are all of you ready for this task?

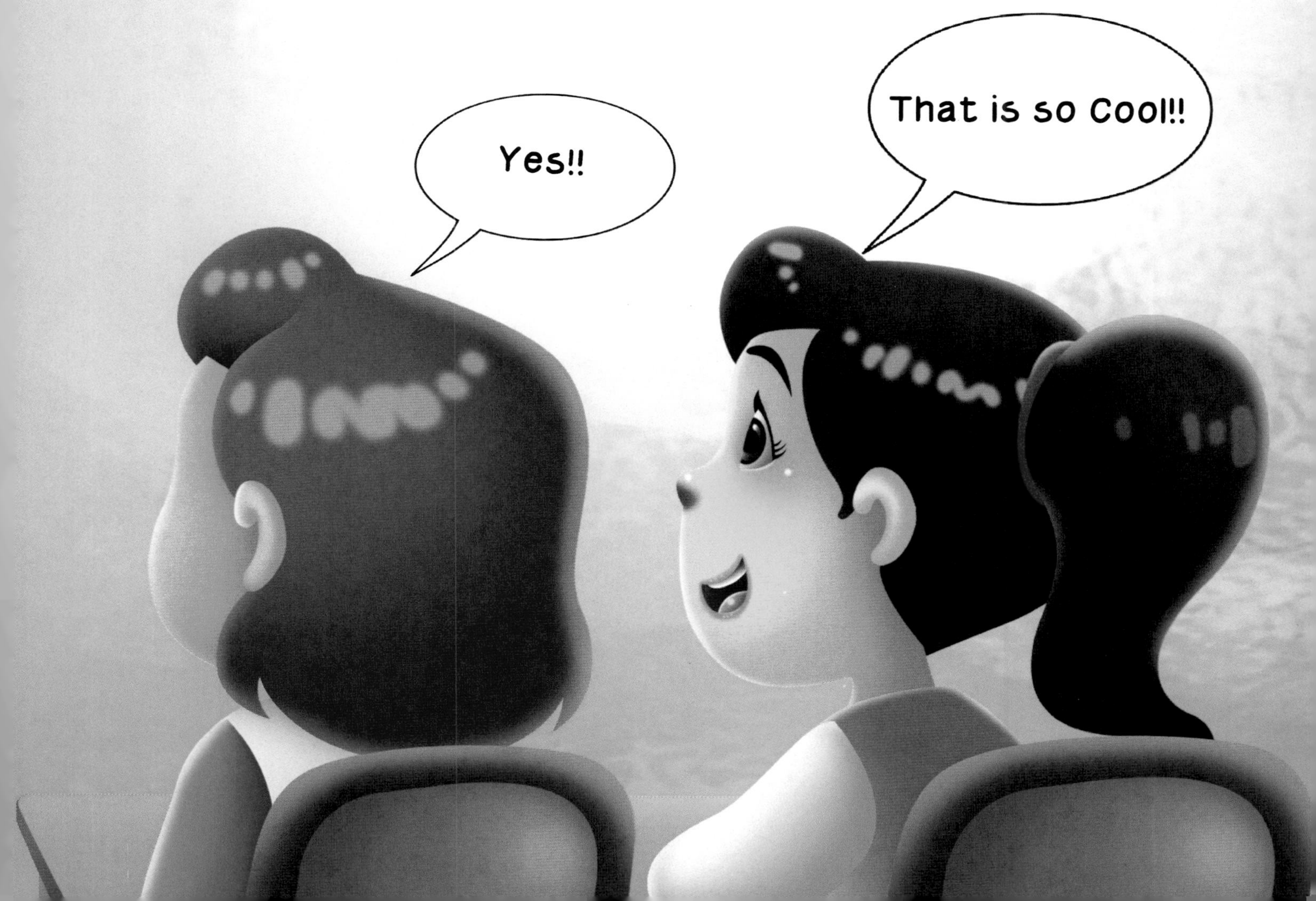
Yes!!
That is so Cool!!

Let's start by using our writing tree,
To help brainstorm ideas for who
your heroes will be.

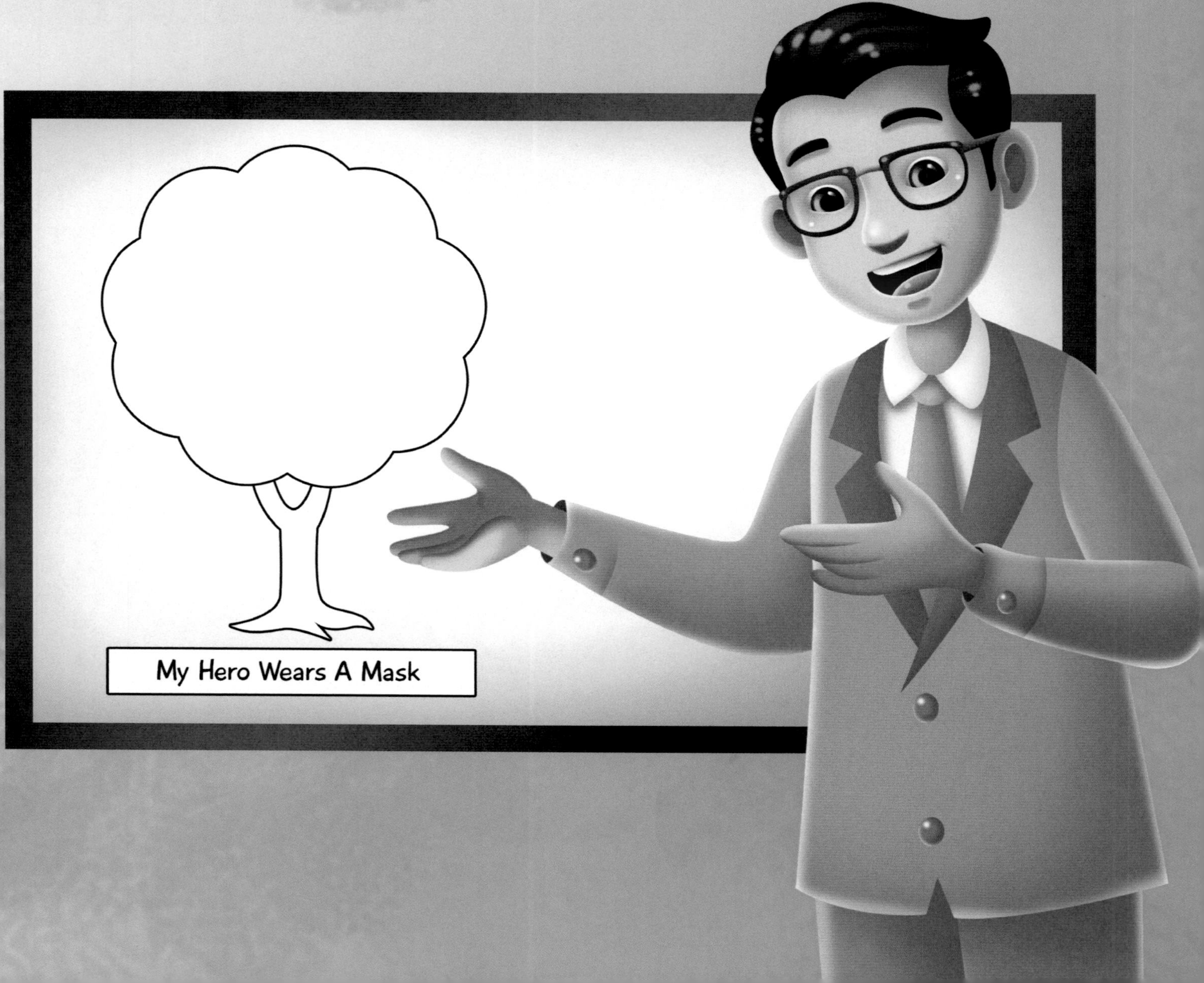
My Hero Wears A Mask

Who would like to go first and share?
Raise your hands so we start to prepare.

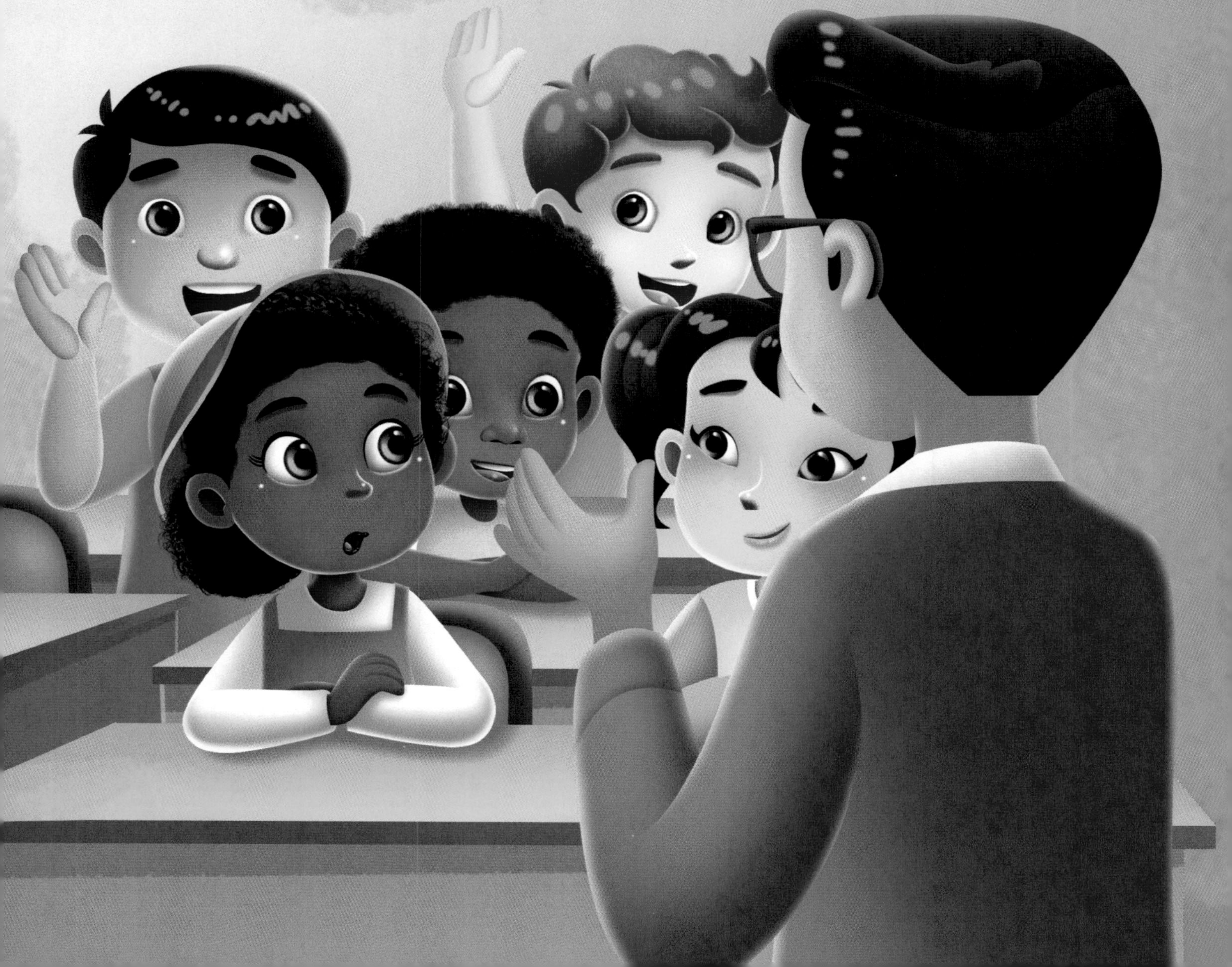

The first few friends yell out, BATMAN! CAT WOMAN! SPIDERMAN!

They are definitely big fans.

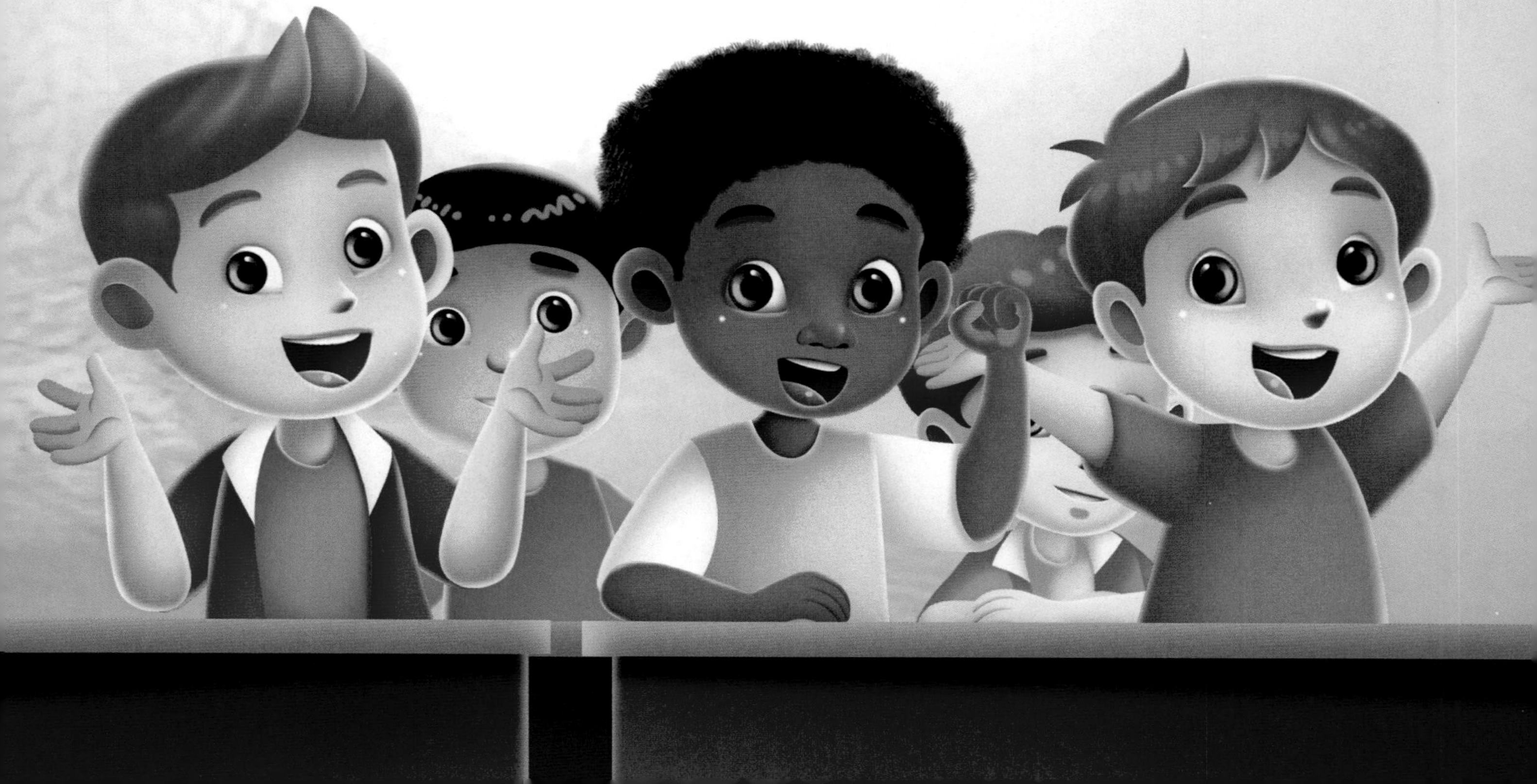

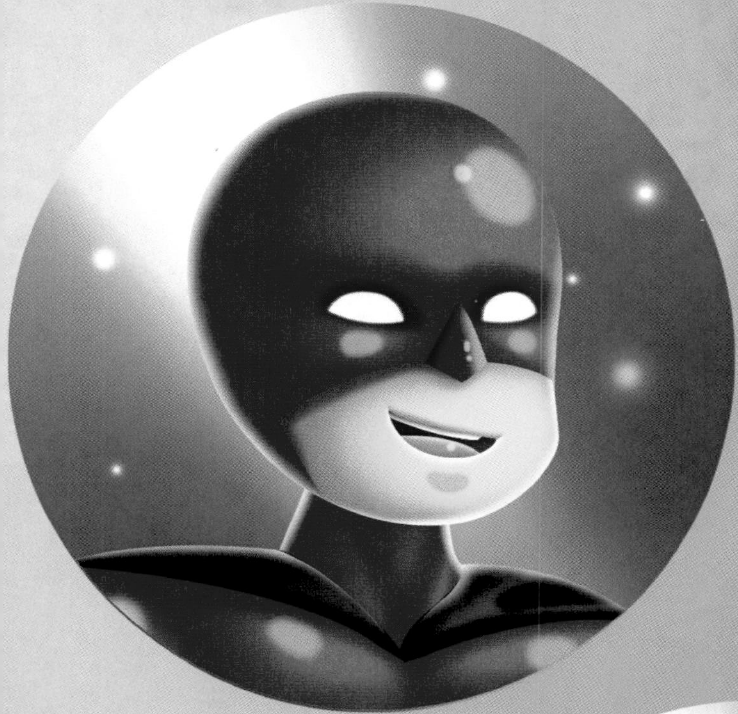
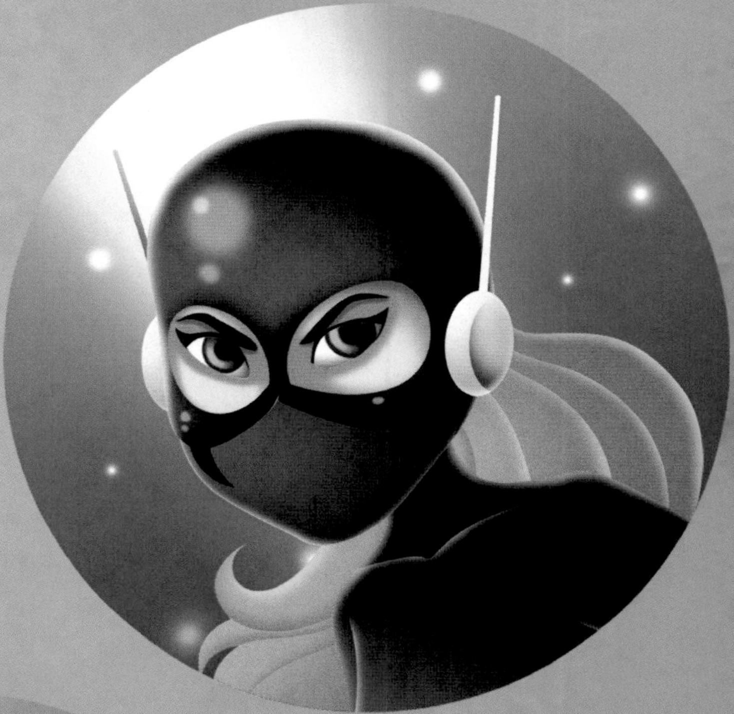
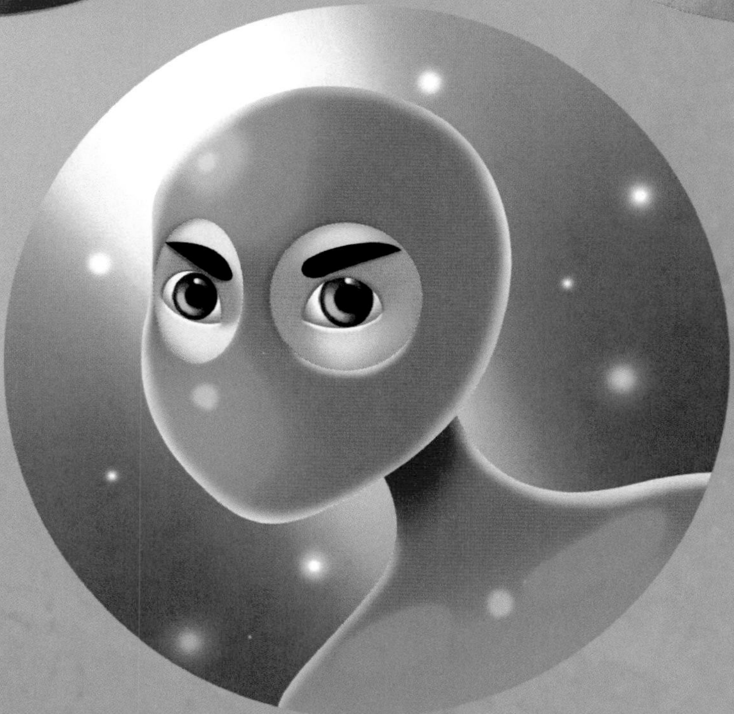

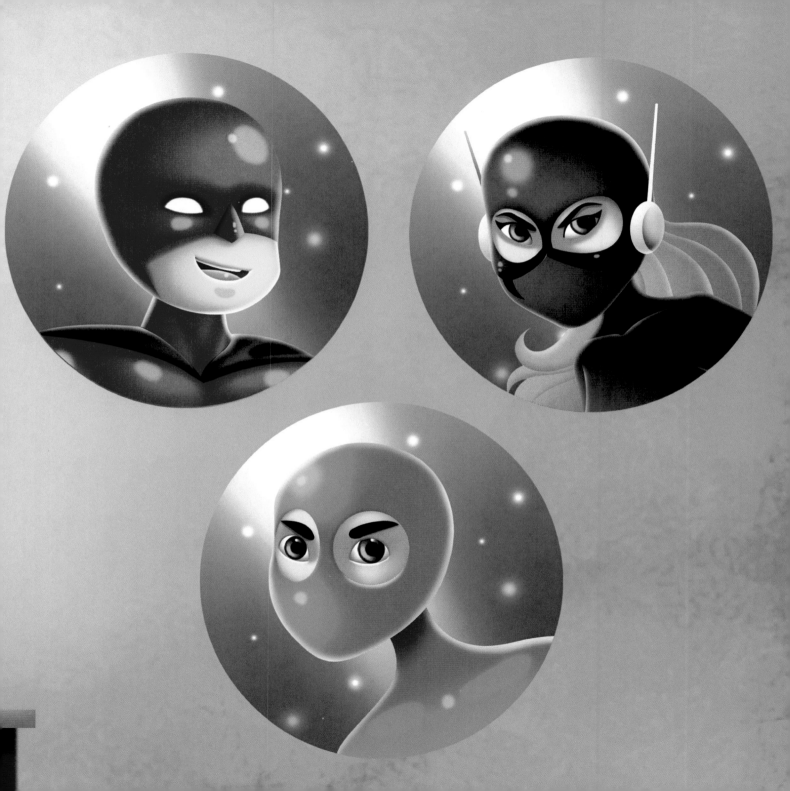

Then it's FIRE FIGHTER! SURGEON! ANESTHESIOLOGIST! DOCTOR! NURSE!

These are frontline workers, their needs come first.

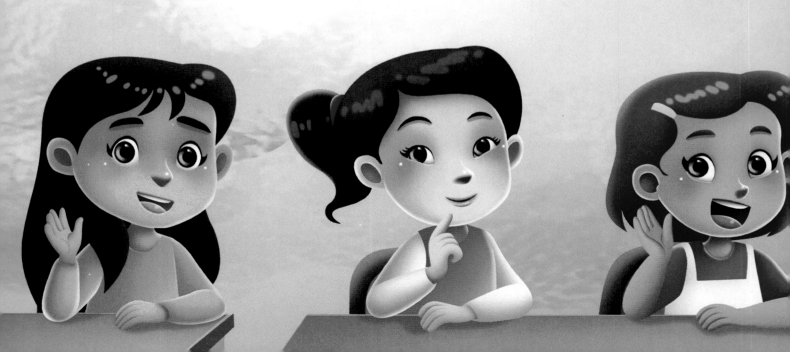

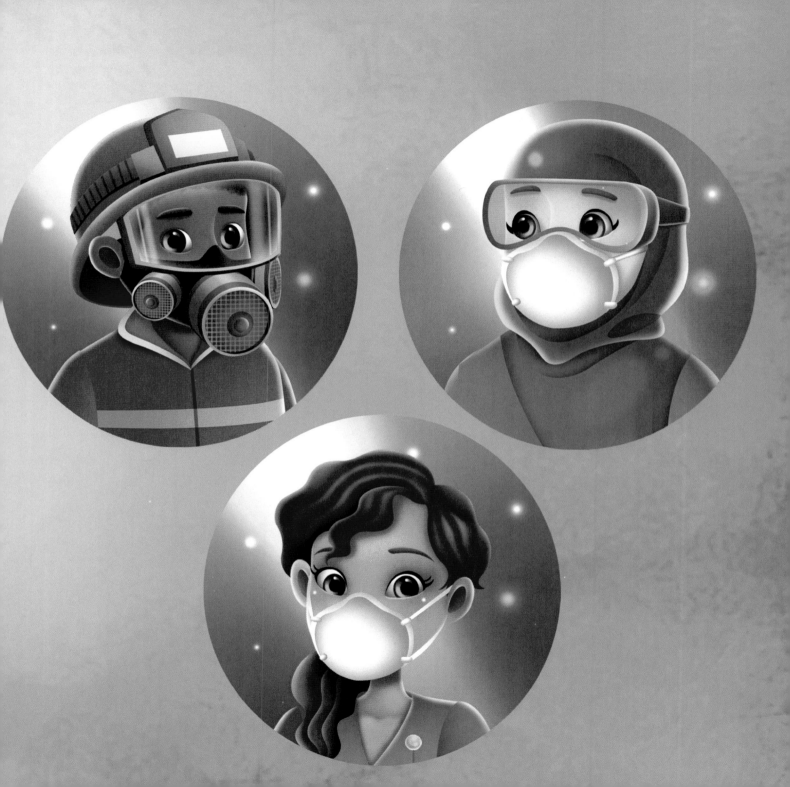

Last but not least, Little Miss chimes in,
"My Hero is my Mom, an Operating Room Nurse."
She teaches everyone about wearing masks so
things do not go from bad to worse.

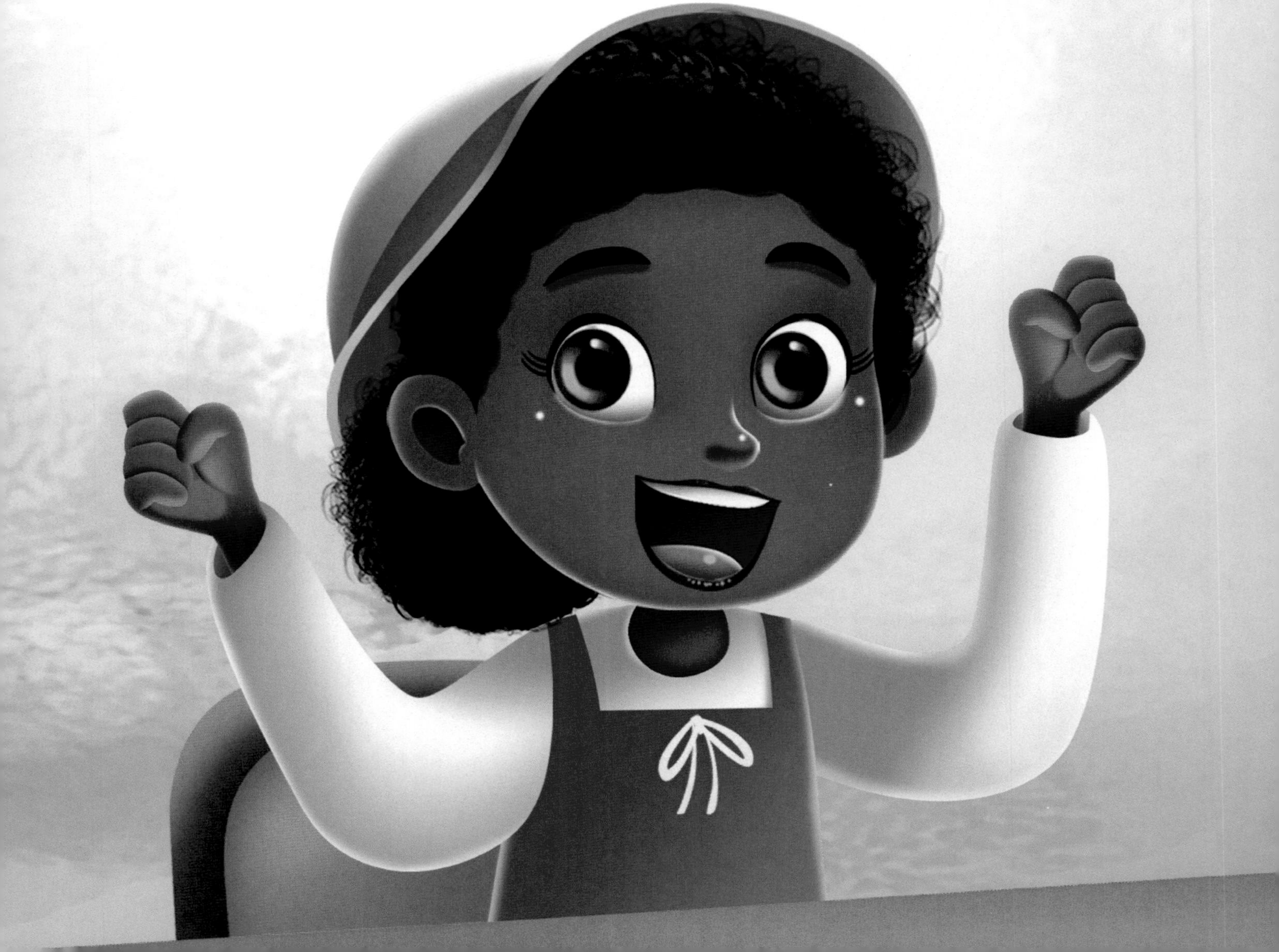

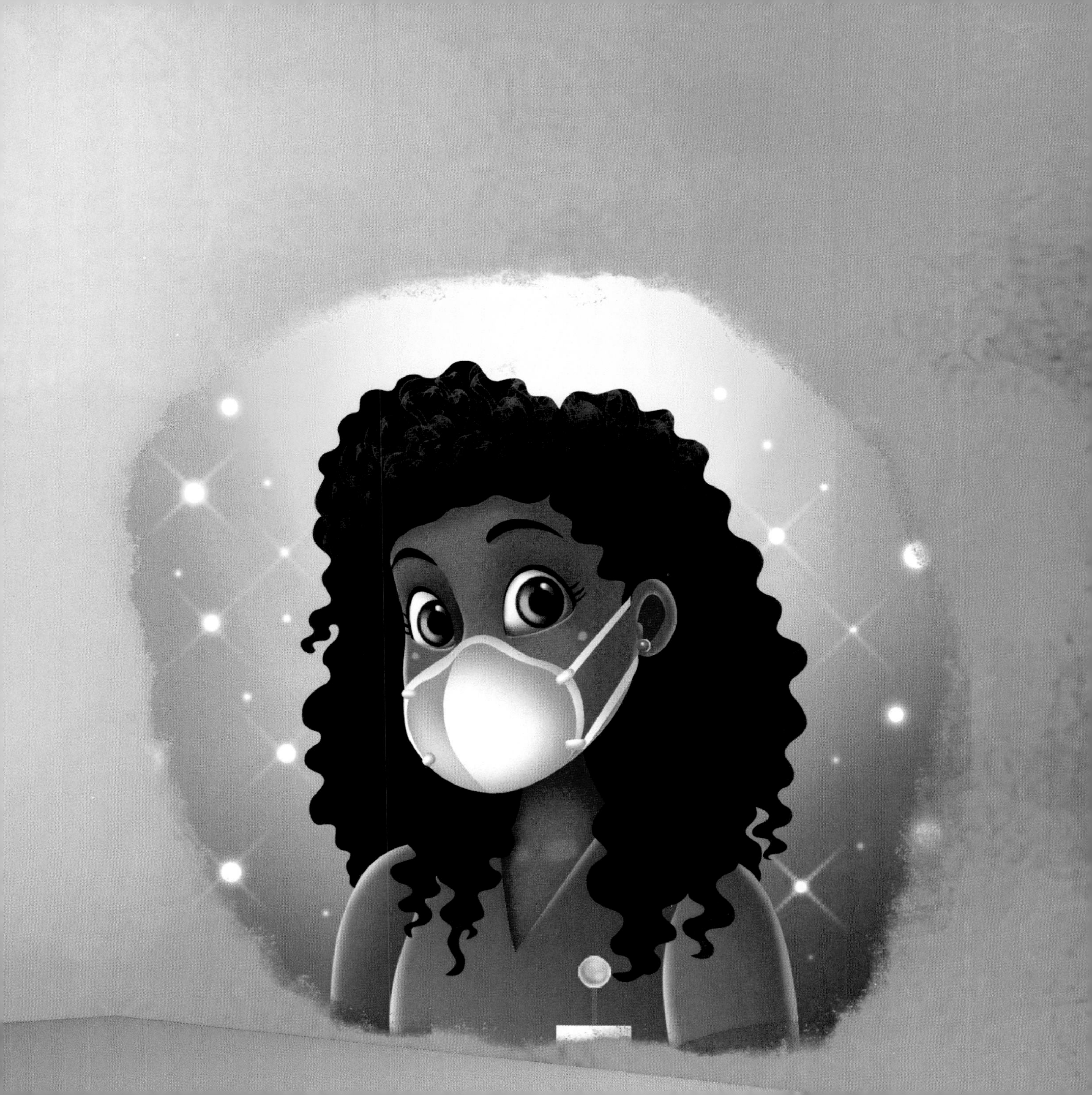

Mr. Jazz reminds us to cover our noses and mouths,
And keep that mask tight, so you do not look like a trout!
Please do not forget to give people their space,
This virus is no joke, so let's just be safe.

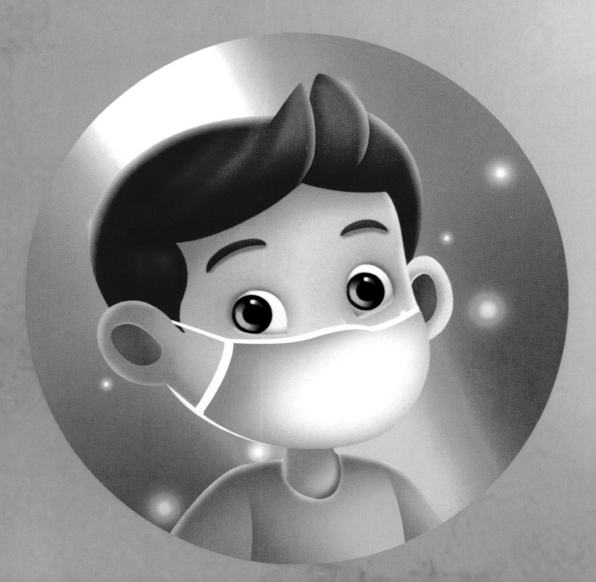

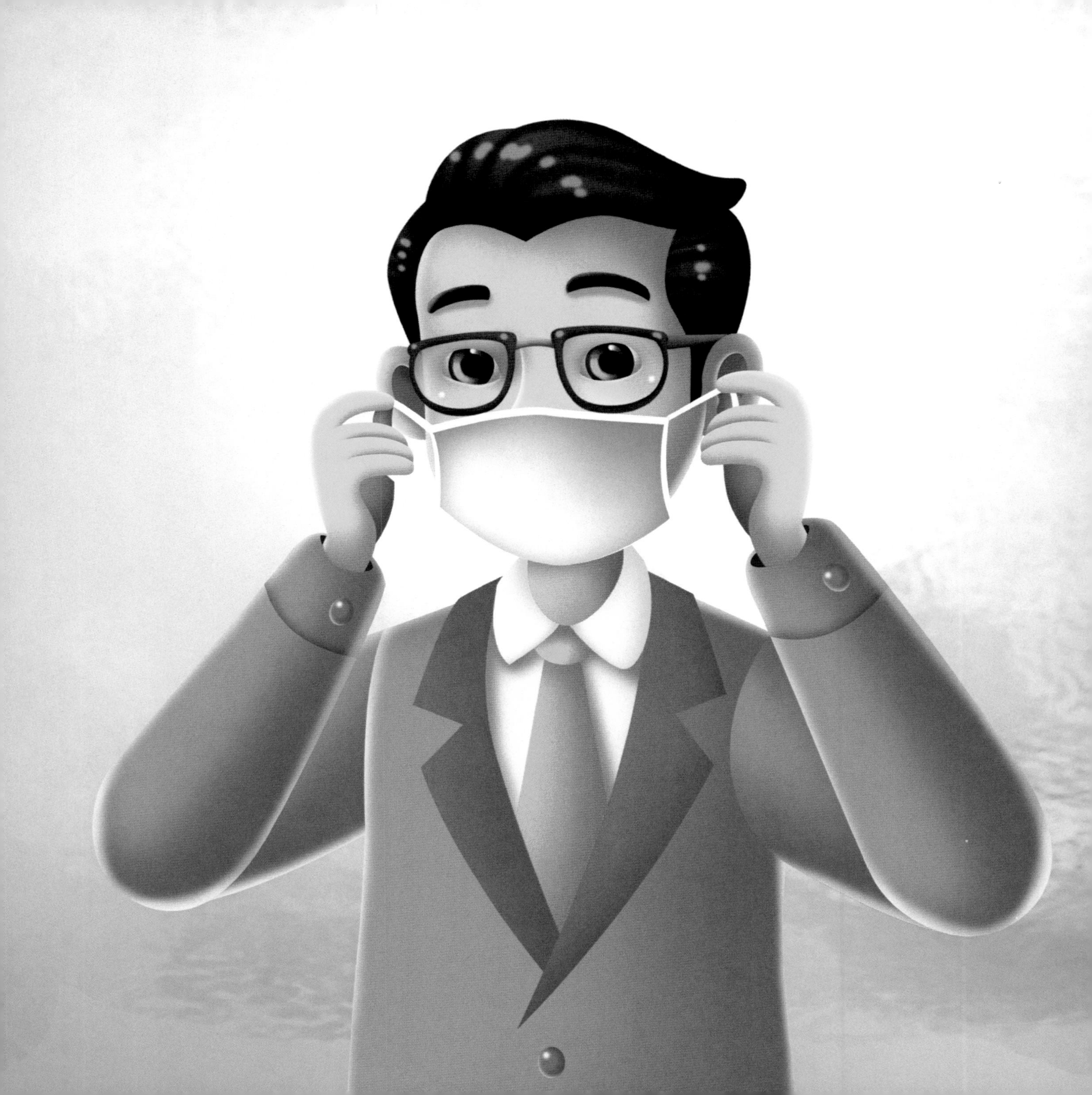

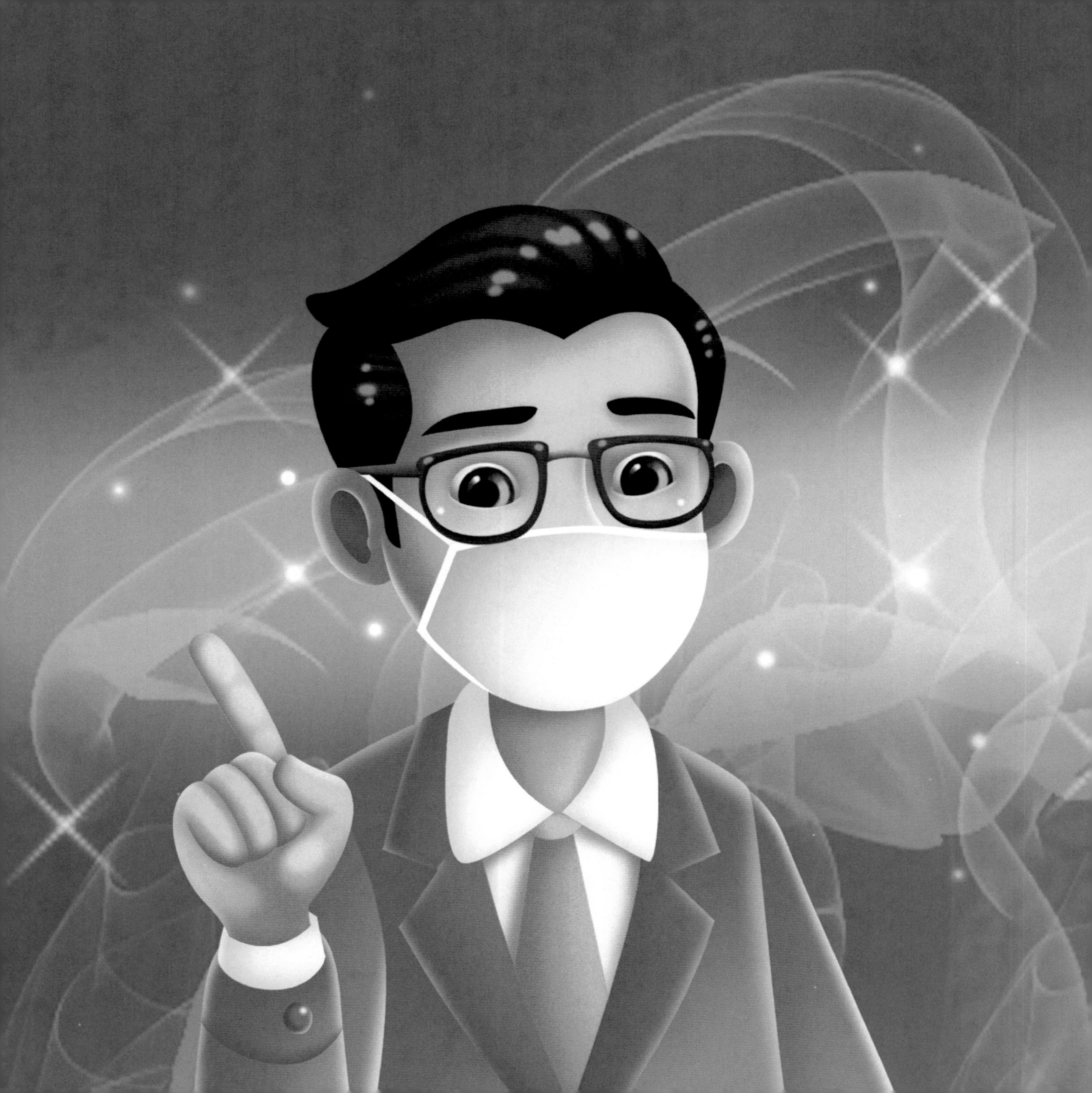

This virus is still such a mystery,
It will definitely go down in history.
We are still learning to stop the spread,
It is just so difficult to keep ahead.

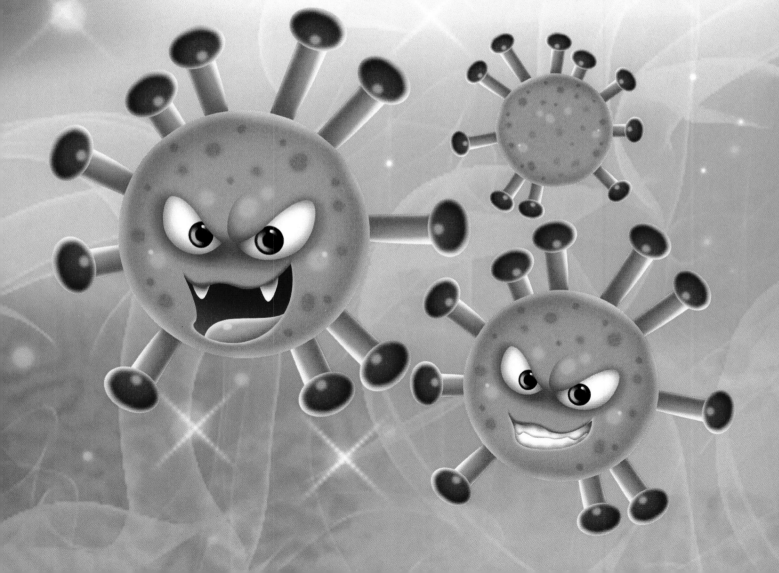

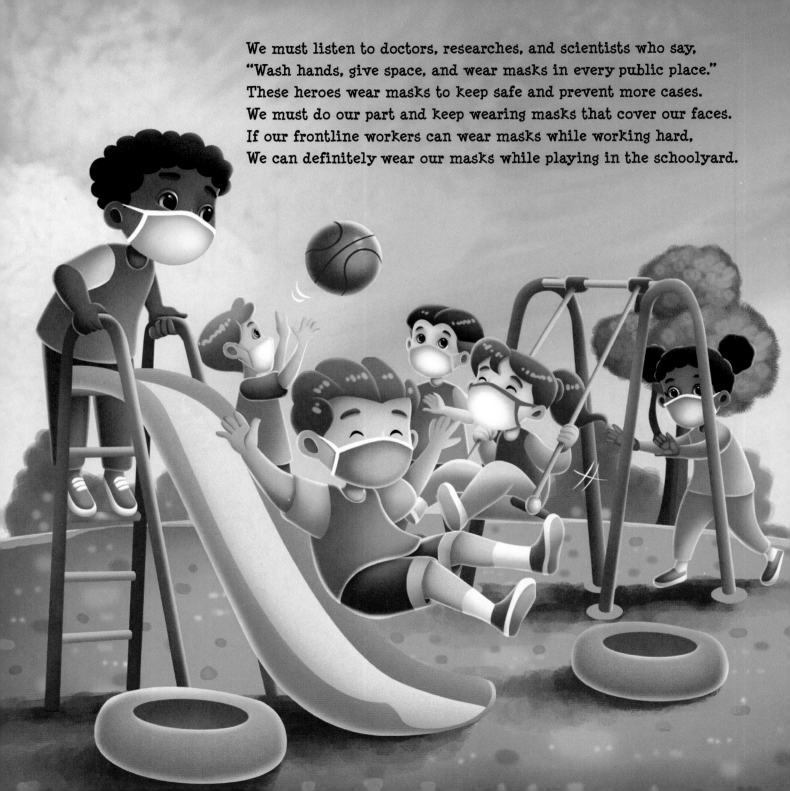

We must listen to doctors, researches, and scientists who say,
"Wash hands, give space, and wear masks in every public place."
These heroes wear masks to keep safe and prevent more cases.
We must do our part and keep wearing masks that cover our faces.
If our frontline workers can wear masks while working hard,
We can definitely wear our masks while playing in the schoolyard.

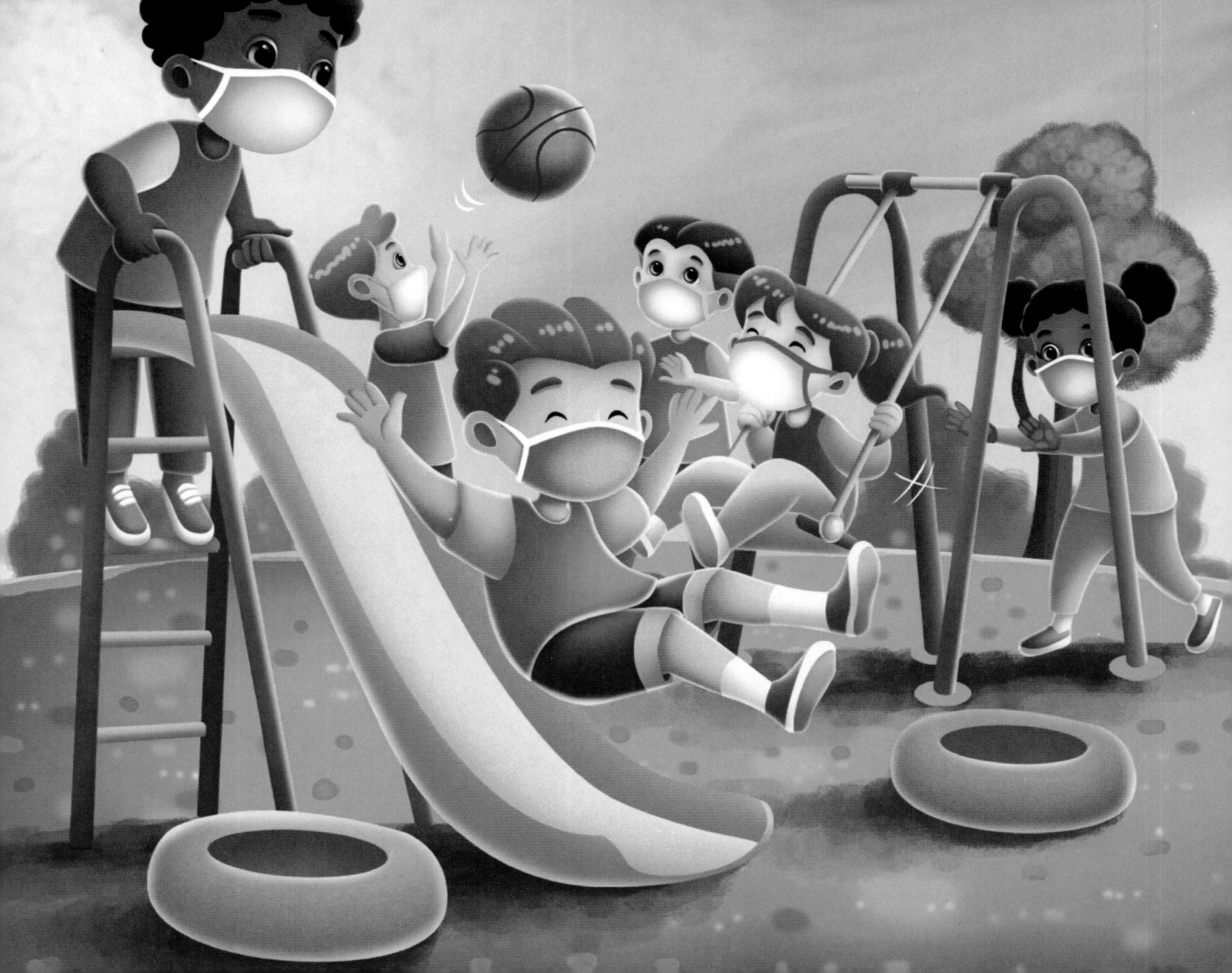

It may be a little hot and stuffy,
But that's nothing compared to frontline workers who are so gutsy.

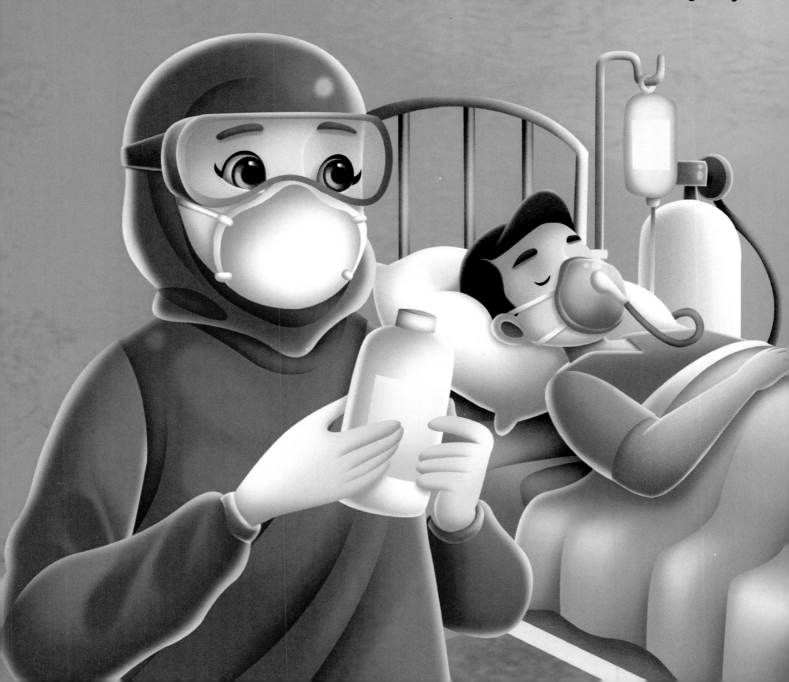

Everyone who wears a mask is a hero.
This helps keep spreading germs close to zero.

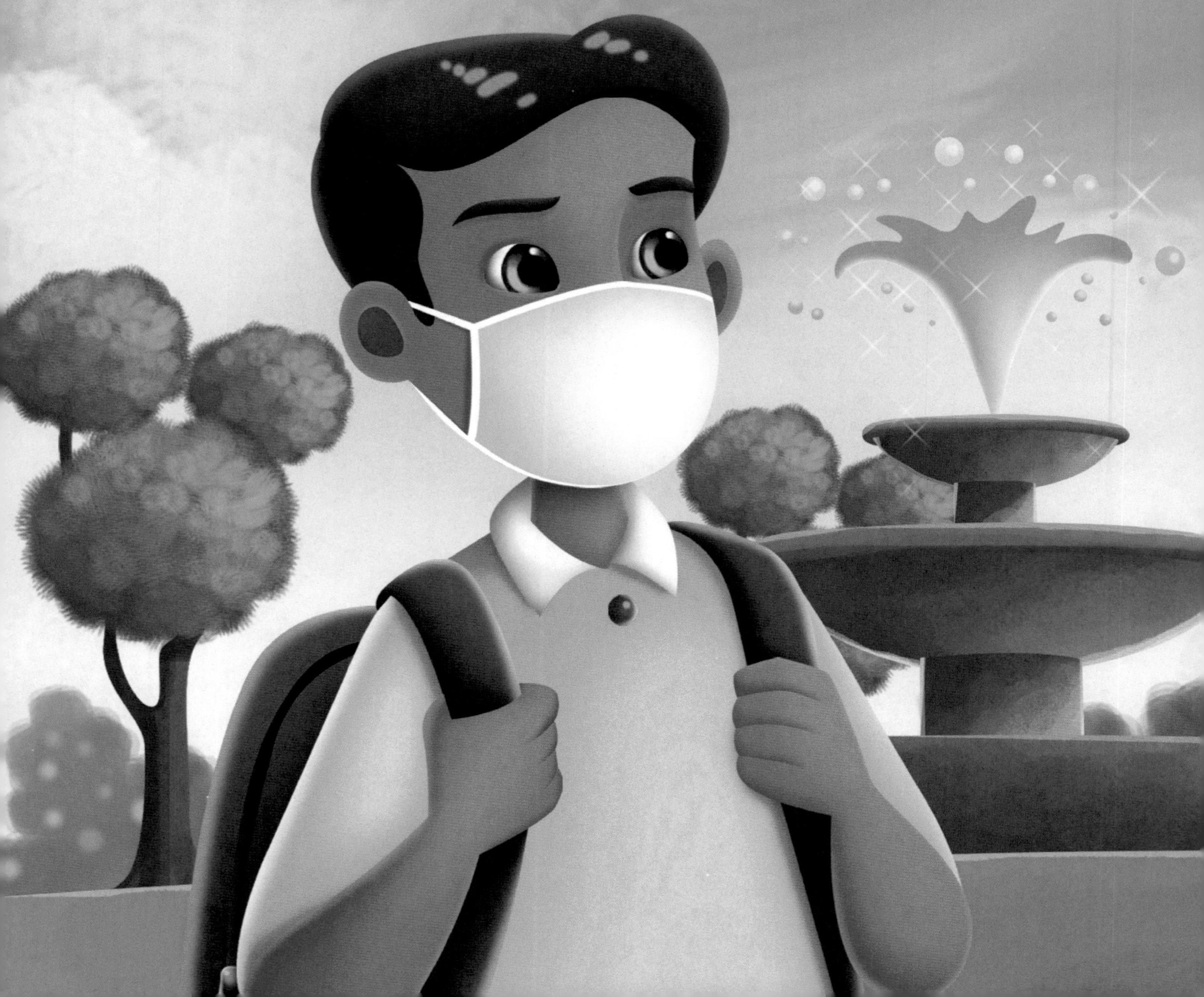

By wearing a mask, you keep everyone around you safe,
Your family, your friends, and your place.

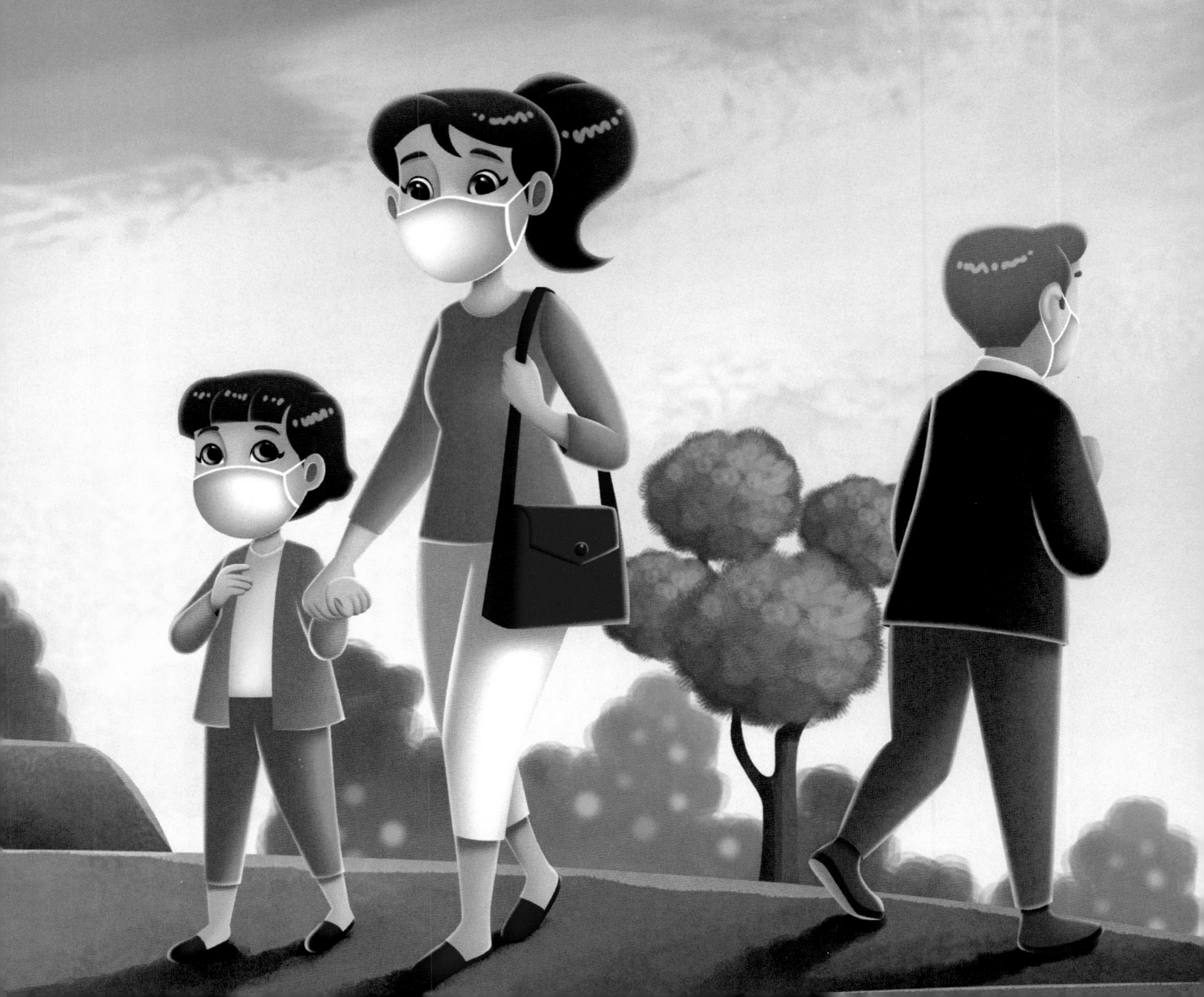

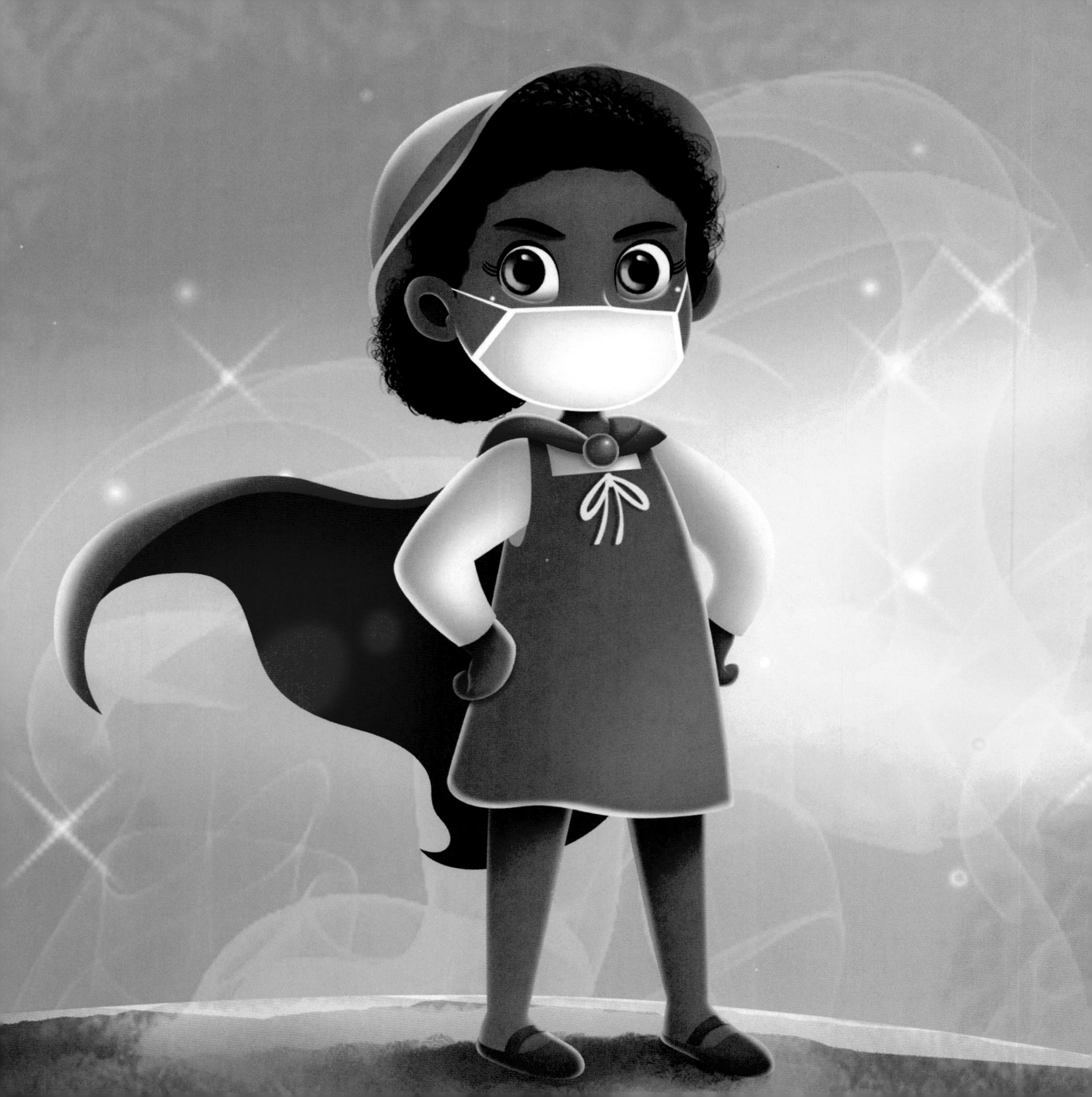

I never thought of it that way,

But by wearing a mask we can save the day!

BE A HERO, WEAR A MASK

It is easy to be super cool like that.

As we get used to our new normal,

Wearing masks, washing hands, and giving space is not abnormal.

Let's all be heroes, and wear our masks,

It is just not that difficult of a task.

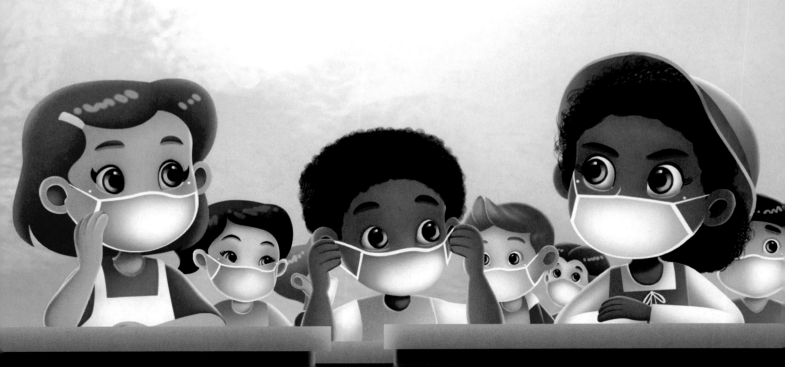

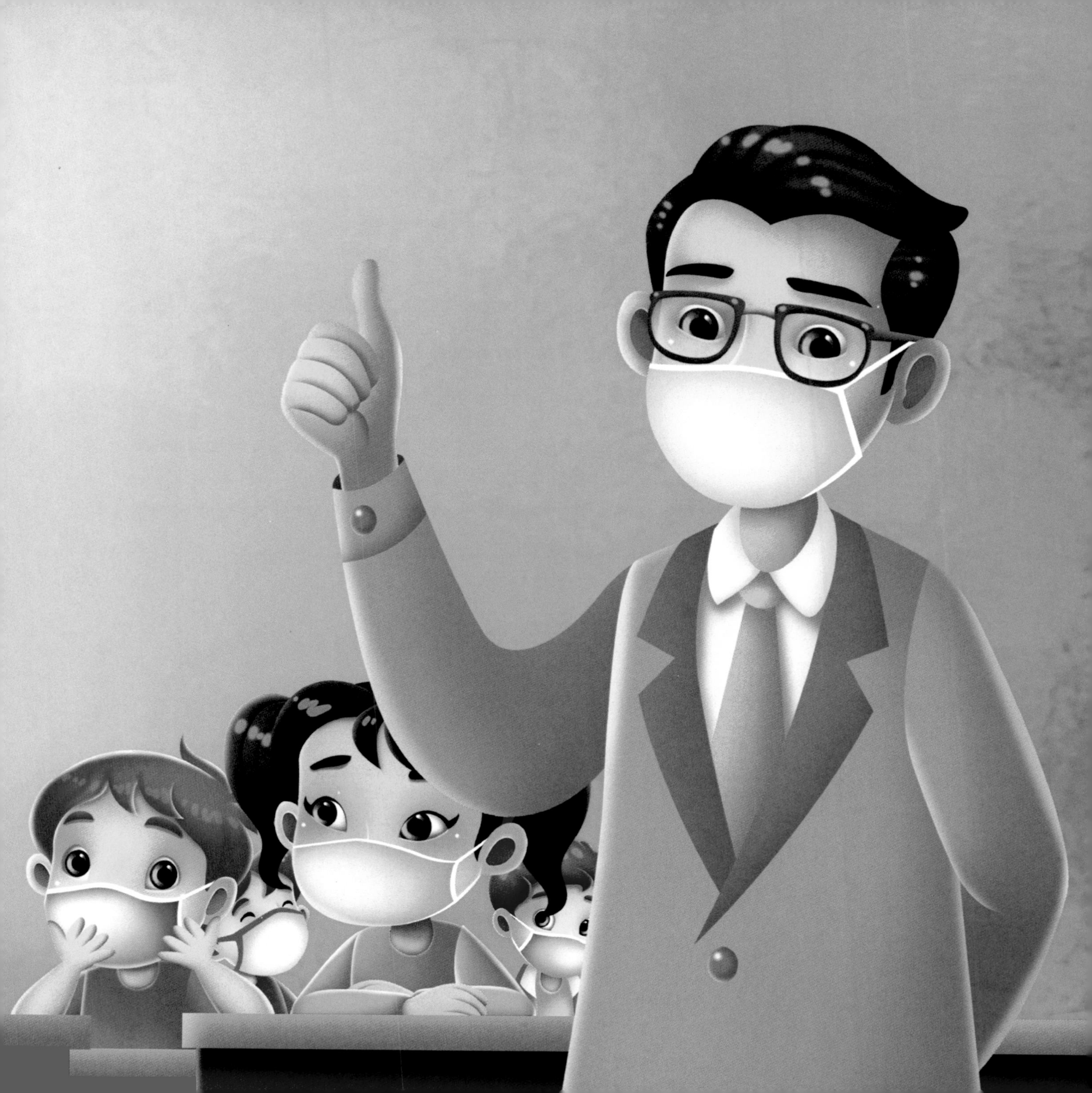

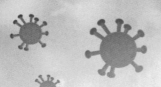

As I write this book COVID 19 has transformed the world as we and our kids know it. Before this book is published, we still do not have a grasp on this pandemic.

The CDC has provided a few essential guidelines for the public to follow to keep ourselves, our families, and community safe.

Wash your hands frequently—especially before eating and after the use of the restroom.

Stand six feet away from others who do not live in the same household.

In public places, wear a mask that covers your nose and mouth

Hand washing is the first line of defense in helping keep ourselves healthy and to stop the spread of germs.

Standing six feet away can help prevent transmission of any germs.

Wearing a mask that covers your nose and mouth helps contain your own germs as well as the germs of others.

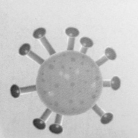

If at all possible, wearing eye shields can also prevent the spread of the virus.

Please keep in mind the many essential workers working every day to ensure that we can continue to live our lives. These essential workers include employees of local hospitals, grocery stores, distribution centers, truck drivers, postal service employees, etc. We honor these individuals with this book.

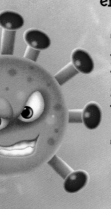

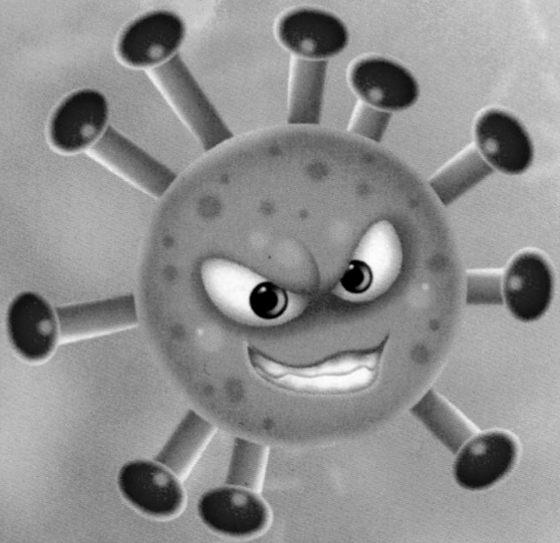

Tell an essential worker today how much you appreciate them. Have your child write them a thank you and teach your kids how to follow the guidelines to protect these essential workers and everyone else in your community.

That's Love,

Erica

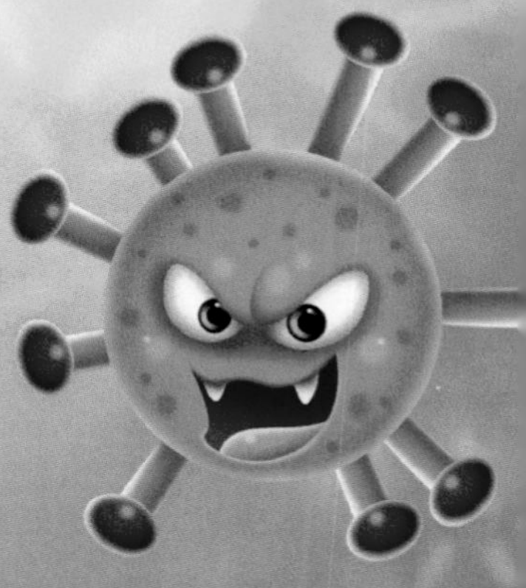

Made in the USA
Middletown, DE
12 May 2022

65667231R00020